COMPLETE GUIDE TO UNDERSTANDING HYSTERECTOMY

Comprehensive Insight, Recovery Strategies For Essential Information, Health Tips, Post-Surgery Care And Emotional Well-Being

KLEIN HOYLE

Disclaimer

The content in this book is based on the author's expertise and comprehension of the topic. The author has no affiliation or link with any corporation, business, or person. This book is meant to give general information and educational material only, and it should not be interpreted as professional medical advice. Always seek the advice of a skilled healthcare expert if you have any queries about medical issues or treatments. The author and publisher expressly disclaim any responsibility resulting directly or indirectly from the use or use of the information included in this book.

ABOUT THIS BOOK

"Complete Guide to Understanding Hysterectomy" provides a thorough guide for anyone navigating the complications of this medical treatment. From explaining the essentials to providing important insights into postoperative living, this book is a beacon of information and support for anybody contemplating or suffering a hysterectomy.

In the first few chapters, readers are introduced to the fundamentals of hysterectomy, including what the process includes, the numerous forms, and the underlying reasons for its need. Individuals may make more educated choices regarding their health by learning about the dangers and advantages of hysterectomy.

Preparation is essential, and Chapter 2 expertly walks readers through the preparation period, from preoperative exams to consultations with healthcare experts. It goes beyond physical preparation to include mental and emotional preparedness, ensuring that patients face surgery with resilience and understanding.

The core of this book is Chapter 3, which describes the many hysterectomy treatments available, ranging from laparoscopic to robotic-assisted approaches. Each strategy is analyzed, providing readers with sophisticated knowledge to help them make decisions.

Recovery is an important step, and Chapter 4 offers a road map for navigating postoperative treatment. From emergency hospital treatment to long-term lifestyle changes, readers are prepared to embark on a path of healing and adaptation.

However, the voyage is not without its hurdles, as discussed in Chapter 5. Individuals are empowered to detect warning symptoms and seek prompt medical attention when information about potential problems and mitigation techniques is provided.

This book goes beyond the physical consequences to explore the hormonal and mental environment after hysterectomy. Chapters 6 and 7 look at the hormonal shifts, menopausal symptoms, and emotional rollercoaster that people may go through, giving comfort and assistance throughout these transitions.

Chapter 8 discusses fertility and family planning, acknowledging the significant influence hysterectomy may have on reproductive choices. Individuals may negotiate this element with clarity and compassion by considering other alternatives and engaging in open talks with partners and healthcare professionals.

Chapter 9 focuses on lifestyle changes and self-care, highlighting the significance of overall well-being after hysterectomy. Readers are inspired to prioritize their health and vitality with tips on everything from food to stress management.

Finally, Chapter 10 marks a fresh beginning, urging readers to reflect on their experience, create objectives, and enjoy life after a hysterectomy. It acts as a light of hope, revealing the many possibilities that await and reinforcing the value of self-care and resilience.

In essence, "Complete Guide to Understanding Hysterectomy" is more than just an instructional resource; it is a companion, confidante, and compass that guides people through the maze of hysterectomy with knowledge, empathy, and empowerment.

CHAPTER 1

Understanding Hysterectomy Basics

What Is A Hysterectomy?

A hysterectomy is a surgical surgery that removes a woman's uterus. This treatment may be partial, removing just a section of the uterus, or complete, removing the whole uterus. Additional reproductive organs, such as the ovaries and fallopian tubes, may be removed based on the individual's medical requirements and the kind of hysterectomy done.

Types Of Hysterectomy Procedures

There are various kinds of hysterectomy surgeries, each with a unique technique and purpose:

1. A complete hysterectomy removes the whole uterus, including the cervix.

This treatment is widely used to treat uterine fibroids, endometriosis, and uterine cancer.

2. A partial hysterectomy, also known as a subtotal or supracervical hysterectomy, is a procedure in which just the top region of the uterus is removed and the cervix is left intact. This surgery may be indicated in situations when maintaining the cervix is regarded helpful.

3. A radical hysterectomy is a more invasive treatment that removes the uterus, cervix, surrounding tissues, and perhaps neighboring lymph nodes. It is often used to treat certain kinds of gynecological malignancies, such as cervical or ovarian cancer.

Reasons To Have A Hysterectomy

A woman may receive a hysterectomy for a variety of reasons, including:

1. Uterine fibroids are noncancerous growths in the uterus that may cause excessive monthly flow, pelvic

discomfort, and pressure on the bladder or intestines. If conservative therapy does not offer relief, a hysterectomy may be indicated.

2. Endometriosis is a disorder in which the tissue that typically lines the lining of the uterus spreads outside of it, causing pelvic discomfort, difficult periods, and reproductive concerns. In extreme situations, a hysterectomy may be required to relieve symptoms.

3. Uterine prolapse occurs when the uterus slides down into the vaginal canal owing to weak pelvic floor muscles. A hysterectomy may be done to address this illness, particularly if other therapies fail.

4. Hysterectomy may be used to treat some forms of gynecological malignancies, such as uterine, cervix, or ovarian cancer. Removing damaged organs may help prevent cancer from spreading to other regions of the body.

Risks And Advantages Of Hysterectomy

Hysterectomy, like any other surgical operation, has risks and advantages that must be carefully weighed.

Benefits:

• Hysterectomy may alleviate symptoms such as persistent pelvic discomfort, irregular bleeding, and other gynecological disorders.

• In gynecological cancer therapy, hysterectomy may lead to remission and better survival chances.

Risks:

• Surgical risks: Hysterectomy is a serious surgery that may cause bleeding, infection, and organ damage.

• Certain types of hysterectomy may cause hormonal changes, leading to menopausal symptoms including hot flashes, mood swings, and vaginal dryness.

• Hysterectomy is a permanent birth control method
that removes the uterus and ovaries. Women who get
a hysterectomy will no longer be able to conceive
naturally.

Individuals seeking a hysterectomy should extensively
examine their choices with their healthcare
professional, weighing the possible risks and
advantages based on their specific circumstances and
medical requirements.

CHAPTER 2

Preparing For Hysterectomy

Preoperative Assessments And Tests

Before having a hysterectomy, your doctor will do many preoperative examinations and tests to verify that you are physically ready for the treatment. These exams assist your healthcare team in understanding your general health and any possible risks related to the procedure.

A thorough analysis of your medical history is one of the major assessments. Your healthcare practitioner will inquire about any existing medical issues, prior operations, drugs you are presently taking, and any allergies you may have. This information is critical for identifying the best anesthetic and surgical technique for your hysterectomy.

In addition, you may have a medical examination to examine your overall health and discover any issues that may compromise the procedure. This checkup usually involves readings of your vital indicators, such as blood pressure, heart rate, and temperature. Your doctor may also do pelvic and abdominal examinations to assess the size and location of your uterus and look for any abnormalities.

In rare situations, you may be required to undertake particular testing before the hysterectomy. These procedures may include blood tests to examine your blood count and clotting function, imaging examinations such as ultrasound or MRI to see your reproductive organs and a Pap smear or biopsy to detect cervical cancer or other abnormalities.

Overall, these preoperative exams and testing are critical to assuring your safety throughout the hysterectomy process. By properly assessing your health state ahead of time, your healthcare team can reduce the chance of problems and adjust the surgical approach to your specific requirements.

Discussing Options With Your Healthcare Provider

Once the preoperative examinations and testing are finished, you should have a thorough conversation with your healthcare physician about the various possibilities for your hysterectomy. This conversation should include a variety of topics, including the surgical strategy, possible risks and advantages, and projected results.

Your healthcare professional will discuss the many kinds of hysterectomy surgeries, such as complete hysterectomy, partial hysterectomy, and radical hysterectomy, and help you decide which one is best for your unique situation. They will also explain if any further surgeries, such as oophorectomy (ovarian removal) or salpingectomy (fallopian tube removal), are required in your situation.

During this talk, you should ask any questions or express any concerns you may have concerning the operation. Your healthcare professional can tell you exactly what to anticipate before, during, and after the hysterectomy, as well as how to manage any possible side effects or problems.

It is also critical to consider the possible effects of the hysterectomy on your fertility and hormone balance, particularly if you are premenopausal. If you are concerned about maintaining fertility, your doctor may advise you on alternate treatment alternatives, such as hormone replacement therapy.

Overall, having an open and honest conversation with your healthcare practitioner about your hysterectomy choices is critical for making educated decisions about your treatment and ensuring that your preferences and concerns are included throughout the process.

Preparing Mentally And Emotionally For Surgery

A hysterectomy may be a life-changing event that elicits a variety of feelings, including worry, fear, grief, and relief. To guarantee a smoother recovery, you must take the time to mentally and emotionally prepare for surgery.

One method to prepare psychologically and emotionally is to learn about the hysterectomy operation and what to anticipate before, during, and after the surgery. This may assist in reducing worry and uncertainty by giving you a better knowledge of the procedure and its results.

Talking with friends or family members who have had a hysterectomy may also be beneficial since they can share their experiences and provide support and encouragement. Consider joining support groups or online forums to connect with people going through similar circumstances and exchange advice and coping skills.

Relaxation methods like deep breathing, meditation, or guided imagery may also help decrease tension and foster a feeling of calm and inner peace in the run-up to surgery. Engaging in enjoyable hobbies, such as reading, listening to music, or spending time outside, may also help you stay optimistic.

Finally, it is important to discuss freely with your healthcare staff about any worries or anxieties you may have before the procedure. They can reassure you, answer your concerns, and give extra support resources if necessary.

By taking proactive actions to psychologically and emotionally prepare for your hysterectomy, you will be able to approach the operation with better confidence and resilience, resulting in a more favorable overall experience and recovery.

Plan For Postoperative Care And Recovery

Following a hysterectomy, good postoperative care and recovery planning are critical for improving healing and reducing complications. Your healthcare practitioner will provide you with specific advice on how to care for yourself after surgery and what to anticipate throughout the recovery period.

Pain and discomfort management is a critical component of postoperative treatment. Your doctor will prescribe pain medicine to assist you in dealing with any discomfort you may encounter after surgery. It is important to take these drugs as prescribed and to tell your healthcare provider if you have any concerns regarding pain management or if your symptoms are not under control.

You will also need to take precautions to aid healing and avoid infection at the surgery site. This may involve keeping the incision clean and dry, changing dressings as appropriate, and refraining from activities that might strain or aggravate the surgical site.

Your healthcare physician will advise you on when it is safe to resume typical activities such as driving, lifting, or exercising, depending on the kind of hysterectomy you had and your healing process. To minimize issues and encourage good recovery, carefully follow these instructions.

In addition to physical recuperation, it is critical to emphasize your mental well-being throughout the postoperative time. As you adapt to life following a hysterectomy, you may feel a variety of feelings, such as relief, grief, or uncertainty. It is important to be patient with oneself and to seek assistance from friends, family members, or mental health specialists as required.

Overall, good postoperative care and recovery planning are critical to a smooth and successful recovery after a hysterectomy.

Following your healthcare provider's recommendations and making efforts to care for your physical and mental well-being can help you recuperate and restore your quality of life after surgery.

CHAPTER 3

Hysterectomy Procedures

Laparoscopic Hysterectomy

Laparoscopic hysterectomy is a minimally invasive surgical technique that removes the uterus via tiny incisions in the abdomen. Many patients and doctors choose this approach over conventional open surgery because it requires less recovery time and has a lower risk of complications.

During a laparoscopic hysterectomy, the surgeon makes numerous tiny incisions in the abdomen, usually around the belly button. A small camera known as a laparoscope is put into one of the incisions, offering a magnified picture of the uterus and surrounding tissues on a monitor in the operating room. Specialized surgical tools are then introduced through the remaining incisions to dissect and remove the uterus.

One benefit of laparoscopic hysterectomy is improved vision of the pelvic organs and tissues, which may lead to more accurate surgical techniques and perhaps less injury to surrounding structures. Furthermore, since the incisions are smaller, there is often less discomfort and scarring following surgery, and patients may recover more quickly than with a standard abdominal hysterectomy.

After the uterus is removed, the surgeon may remove the ovaries and fallopian tubes if required. This procedure is characterized as a complete laparoscopic hysterectomy with bilateral salpingo-oophorectomy.

Overall, laparoscopic hysterectomy is a less intrusive option to standard open surgery that may result in shorter hospital stays, quicker recovery periods, and fewer problems.

Abdominal Hysterectomy

Abdominal hysterectomy is a surgical technique that removes the uterus via a wider incision in the abdomen. While it is more intrusive than laparoscopic or vaginal hysterectomy, it may be essential in certain circumstances, such as when the uterus is particularly big or there are other complications.

During an abdominal hysterectomy, the physician makes a single incision in the lower abdomen, often at the bikini line. This incision opens up the uterus and enables the surgeon to physically evaluate the pelvic organs and surrounding tissues.

After exposing the uterus, the surgeon gently separates it from the surrounding tissues and blood arteries before removing it from the body. The ovaries and fallopian tubes may be removed during the treatment, depending on the patient's medical history and the cause of the hysterectomy.

While abdominal hysterectomy is often linked with a lengthier recovery time and a greater risk of complications than less invasive methods such as laparoscopic or vaginal hysterectomy, it may be the best choice for certain individuals. Women with big fibroids or significant endometriosis, for example, may need an abdominal hysterectomy to guarantee that the uterus and surrounding tissues are fully removed.

After surgery, patients should expect to spend several days in the hospital healing before being sent home. An abdominal hysterectomy might take many weeks to completely recover, therefore patients should avoid heavy lifting and intense activities to enable the incision to heal correctly.

Vaginal Hysterectomy

A vaginal hysterectomy is a surgical treatment that removes the uterus via the vagina without creating exterior incisions in the abdomen. This method has various potential advantages, including shorter recovery periods, fewer problems, and no visible scarring.

A vaginal hysterectomy involves the surgeon making a tiny incision within the vagina and using specialized equipment to separate the uterus from the surrounding ligaments and blood vessels. The uterus is then delicately removed from the body via the vagina.

Vaginal hysterectomy is often chosen for individuals with particular medical issues, such as uterine prolapse or irregular uterine bleeding, since the uterus may be readily reached and removed via the vaginal canal. It may also be indicated for women who want to avoid abdominal incisions or have a history of abdominal surgery, which raises the risk of problems.

Because there are no external incisions, healing from vaginal hysterectomy is usually quicker than from abdominal hysterectomy. Most patients may go home the same day or the day following surgery and return to regular activities within a few weeks.

However, it is critical to follow your surgeon's postoperative care guidelines and avoid heavy lifting or intense activities until completely recovered.

Robotic Assisted Hysterectomy

Robotic-assisted hysterectomy is a minimally invasive surgical treatment that removes the uterus using the accuracy of robotic technology and the expertise of a skilled physician. Compared to conventional open surgery, this method has the potential to result in smaller incisions, shorter hospital stays, and quicker recovery periods.

During a robotic-assisted hysterectomy, the surgeon sits at a console in the operating room and directs robotic arms carrying surgical equipment. These devices are placed via tiny incisions in the belly, enabling the surgeon to execute the treatment with more accuracy and skill.

The surgeon employs a high-definition 3D camera to offer a magnified, high-resolution picture of the surgical site, enabling more accurate dissection and removal of the uterus and surrounding tissues. This may lead to less blood loss, lower complications, and shorter recovery periods for patients.

Robotic-assisted hysterectomy may be indicated for individuals with certain medical problems, such as big fibroids or widespread endometriosis when robotic technology's accuracy and dexterity might give additional advantages. It may also be preferable for individuals who are ineligible for standard laparoscopic surgery owing to anatomical limitations or prior abdominal surgery.

Patients should anticipate to stay in the hospital for a short period after surgery before being released. Most patients feel less pain and discomfort than with typical open surgery, and they may return to regular activities within a few weeks.

To ensure a smooth recovery, you should follow your surgeon's postoperative care recommendations and attend follow-up consultations.

CHAPTER 4

Recovery And Aftercare

Immediate Postoperative Care At The Hospital

Following a hysterectomy, you will be carefully followed in the hospital for any symptoms of problems or pain. Your medical team will make sure you're stable and comfortable as you recuperate from surgery. This phase is critical for your health and lays the groundwork for a healthy recovery process.

When you wake up from anesthesia, you may feel groggy, nauseated, or uncomfortable. Your healthcare experts will respond quickly to these symptoms to guarantee your comfort. They will also check your vital indicators, such as blood pressure, heart rate, and respiration, to make sure you are stable.

You can have a catheter in place to assist drain pee from your bladder. This is temporary and will be removed once you can urinate independently. You may also wear a bandage over the incision site to prevent infection. Your healthcare team will change the dressing as appropriate and keep an eye on the incision for symptoms of infection or problems.

Throughout your hospital stay, you will be given pain medicine to assist you manage any discomfort. It is important to talk freely with your medical team about your pain levels so that they can alter your medication accordingly. They will also advise you on how to move and arrange yourself carefully to avoid pressure on your incision site.

During this time, your medical staff will also give you advice on what to eat and drink. Follow these suggestions to help your body recuperate and avoid issues like constipation and dehydration.

Manage Pain And Discomfort At Home

Once you are released from the hospital, controlling pain and discomfort at home becomes a top priority in your rehabilitation. To assist reduce pain, your healthcare team will prescribe medicine, which must be taken exactly as prescribed.

In addition to medicine, there are numerous ways to manage pain and discomfort at home. Ice packs may help decrease swelling and numbness around the incision site. To avoid frostbite, place a cloth or towel between the ice pack and your skin.

Getting lots of rest is also important at this time. Listen to your body and take pauses when necessary, even if it means changing your regular schedule or asking for assistance with domestic activities. Avoid lifting heavy things or indulging in physical exercise until your healthcare practitioner gives you the go-ahead.

Maintaining proper nourishment and water is critical for your body's healing process. Consume a balanced diet high in fruits, vegetables, lean proteins, and whole grains. Drink lots of water throughout the day to keep hydrated and support proper recovery.

Resuming Daily Activities And Exercise

As you feel better, you may want to resume your usual daily activities and exercise program. To avoid injury or difficulties, you should start slowly and gradually raise your exercise level.

Begin by introducing simple exercises like walking or easy stretching into your routine. Listen to your body and stop if you feel pain or discomfort. As your strength and endurance improve, you may progressively increase the intensity and length of your exercises.

Avoid high-impact activities and heavy lifting until your doctor gives you the go-ahead. Concentrate on activities that strengthen the core muscles and improve flexibility and stability. Consider working with a physical therapist to create a safe and effective fitness regimen that is specific to your requirements.

Long-Term Effects And Lifestyle Adjustments

While a hysterectomy may help with some medical concerns, it's important to understand the long-term repercussions and lifestyle changes that may result from the treatment. For example, some women may develop hormonal imbalances, resulting in symptoms such as hot flashes, mood swings, or vaginal dryness.

It is important to share any concerns or questions you have regarding the long-term consequences with your healthcare professional. They may help you manage your symptoms and adapt to life after having a hysterectomy.

They may also offer hormone replacement therapy or other therapies to aid with symptom management and quality of life.

In terms of lifestyle changes, it's critical to listen to your body and emphasize self-care. Set aside time for relaxation and stress-management practices including meditation, yoga, and deep breathing exercises. Surround yourself with a supportive group of friends and family who can give encouragement and aid when required.

Overall, recovery following a hysterectomy requires patience, self-care, and an openness to your body's demands. Following your healthcare provider's advice and making efforts to support your physical and mental well-being can help you traverse the recovery process with confidence and resilience.

CHAPTER 5

Possible Complications

Surgical Risks And Possible Complications

Hysterectomy, like other surgeries, has risks and consequences. Understanding the hazards is critical for anybody contemplating or going through the treatment.

1. Infection: Any surgical operation has the danger of infection. Your surgeon will take precautions to reduce this risk, such as giving antibiotics before and after surgery and keeping strict sterile conditions in the operating room. If an infection does develop, it is typically treatable with medications.

2. Bleeding may occur during or after surgery. Your surgeon will take precautions to reduce bleeding

during the surgery, but severe bleeding may need extra treatment or possibly a blood transfusion.

3. Blood Clots: Following surgery, blood clots may develop in the legs (deep vein thrombosis) or migrate to the lungs (pulmonary embolism). To lessen this risk, you may be given blood thinners and advised to walk about as soon as possible following surgery.

4. Injury to adjoining organs: During a hysterectomy, nearby organs such as the bladder or intestines may be accidently harmed. This is uncommon, but it may occur. Your surgeon will take precautions to prevent such accidents, but you should be aware of the possibilities.

5. Anesthesia dangers: There are risks associated with anesthesia, such as allergic responses and problems. Your anesthesiologist will review your medical history and take action to reduce the risks.

How To Prevent Complications

While problems are always a possibility following surgery, there are things you may do to lessen your chances of encountering them:

1. **Follow pre-operative instructions:** Before your surgery, your surgeon will give you particular directions to follow, such as not taking certain medicines or fasting for a certain amount of time. Following these steps attentively may help lessen the likelihood of difficulties.

2. **Maintain a healthy lifestyle:** Eating a well-balanced diet, exercising frequently, and quitting smoking may improve your general health and lower your chance of problems before and after surgery.

3. **Communicate with your healthcare team:** Make sure to communicate any concerns or questions you have with your surgeon and the rest of your healthcare

team. They may provide information and assistance to help reduce the likelihood of issues.

Identifying Signs Of Complications

Even with careful planning and procedures, difficulties might arise. It's important to recognize the indicators of possible problems so that you may seek immediate medical assistance if necessary.

1. Symptoms of infection include fever, redness, warmth, and increasing discomfort at the surgical site. If you see any of these symptoms, call your doctor straight away.

2. **Excessive bleeding:** Some bleeding is typical after surgery, but if you have severe bleeding that does not stop with rest and elevation, or if you pass big clots, get medical assistance right once.

3. **Difficulty breathing:** Shortness of breath or chest discomfort may indicate a blood clot in the lungs

(pulmonary embolism), requiring emergency medical intervention.

4. Severe pain: While some discomfort is normal after surgery, severe or increasing pain may suggest a problem such as organ damage or infection.

Seeking Prompt Medical Attention, If Needed

If you have any symptoms or indicators of problems after your hysterectomy, do not hesitate to seek medical assistance. Early management may frequently save issues from worsening and result in a faster recovery. If you are concerned about your recuperation, contact your surgeon or visit the local emergency facility. Your healthcare staff is there to help you and keep you safe throughout the procedure.

CHAPTER 6

Hormonal Changes And Menopause

Effects Of Hysterectomy On Hormone Balance

When having a hysterectomy, it is critical to understand how the treatment will affect your hormonal balance. The removal of the uterus may have a substantial impact on hormone production and control in your body, especially if the ovaries are also removed during surgery.

The uterus helps regulate hormones, especially during menstruation. Its removal may upset the body's normal hormonal balance, causing fluctuations in hormone levels. If the ovaries remain intact, they may continue to generate hormones such as estrogen and progesterone, but in differing proportions than previously.

However, removing the ovaries (a technique known as bilateral oophorectomy) results in a sudden beginning of menopause. The ovaries are the principal source of estrogen and progesterone in premenopausal women. Without them, hormone levels plummet, resulting in symptoms including hot flashes, mood swings, vaginal dryness, and reduced libido.

The level of hormonal alterations after a hysterectomy varies based on age, general health, and whether or not the ovaries are removed. Younger women who have hysterectomy without oophorectomy may have fewer hormonal abnormalities than those who have their ovaries removed.

Before having a hysterectomy, you should talk to your doctor about the possible hormonal side effects. They may provide you with tailored advice based on your medical history and explain what to anticipate with hormonal changes.

Managing Menopausal Symptoms After A Hysterectomy

Managing menopausal symptoms after hysterectomy is an important part of postoperative treatment. Menopause may occur suddenly after the removal of the uterus and/or ovaries, causing a variety of painful symptoms that damage your quality of life.

Hot flashes are a common symptom, which are abrupt sensations of warmth that are often accompanied by perspiration and flushing of the face and neck. These may be controlled with lifestyle adjustments such as wearing breathable clothes, avoiding spicy foods and caffeine, and practicing relaxation methods such as deep breathing or meditation.

Another common symptom is vaginal dryness, which may be uncomfortable during intercourse and raises the risk of urinary tract infections. Using over-the-counter vaginal lubricants or moisturizers may aid with this discomfort and general comfort.

Mood swings and irritability are also frequent throughout menopause, and developing good coping strategies like regular exercise, social support, and stress management skills may help manage these emotional shifts.

Furthermore, some women may report a reduction in libido or sexual desire after hysterectomy-induced menopause. Open discussion with your spouse and exploring different types of closeness might help you maintain a satisfying sexual relationship despite these changes.

Hormone replacement treatment (HRT) may be used if symptoms are severe or have a major effect on everyday life. HRT is taking estrogen and occasionally progesterone to replace hormones that your body no longer generates naturally. However, it is important to explore the dangers and advantages of HRT with your doctor, since it may not be appropriate for everyone.

Hormone Replacement Therapy Options

Hormone replacement therapy (HRT) is a frequent treatment for menopausal symptoms after hysterectomy. It entails replenishing hormones that your body no longer generates naturally owing to the removal of the uterus and/or ovaries.

There are two forms of HRT available: estrogen-only treatment (ET) and combination estrogen-progestin therapy (EPT). ET is often suggested for women who have had a hysterectomy since they no longer have a uterus and so do not need progesterone to prevent uterine cancer.

EPT, on the other hand, is suggested for women who still have a uterus since it contains both estrogen and progesterone, reducing the risk of endometrial cancer associated with estrogen treatment alone.

HRT may be taken in a variety of ways, including tablets, patches, creams, gels, and sprays. Personal taste, convenience, and individual health concerns all influence the type of administration used.

Before beginning HRT therapy, you must consider the risks and benefits with your doctor. HRT may successfully relieve menopausal symptoms, but it is not without hazards. Long-term usage of HRT has been linked to an increased risk of certain health problems, such as breast cancer, heart disease, and blood clots.

Your healthcare professional can assist you in weighing the risks and advantages of HRT depending on your specific medical history, symptoms, and preferences. They may also track your progress and make any required changes to your treatment plan to safeguard your overall health and well-being.

Discussing Long-Term Health Implications With Your Doctor

When having a hysterectomy, you should address the long-term health concerns with your doctor. While the technique is successful in treating specific medical disorders, it is not without dangers and repercussions.

One of the biggest concerns with hysterectomy is the effect on bone health. Estrogen is essential for maintaining bone density, and a fast decline in estrogen levels during hysterectomy-induced menopause might raise the risk of osteoporosis and bone fractures.

To reduce this risk, your doctor may suggest lifestyle modifications such as regular weight-bearing activity, calcium and vitamin D supplements, and quitting smoking and excessive alcohol intake.

Another factor to consider is the possibility of developing cardiovascular disease.

Estrogen protects the cardiovascular system, and a lack of estrogen after hysterectomy may raise the risk of heart disease and stroke. Your doctor may evaluate your cardiovascular risk factors and propose lifestyle changes or drugs to lower your risk.

Furthermore, it is critical to examine the possible effects of hysterectomy on sexual function and pelvic floor health. Some women may have changes in sexual feelings or pelvic organ prolapse after the treatment; your doctor may advise you on how to manage these difficulties while maintaining sexual function and pelvic floor integrity.

Overall, honest discussion with your doctor is essential for understanding the long-term health consequences of hysterectomy and building an effective post-operative treatment and follow-up plan. Working together may help you achieve maximum health and well-being in the years after surgery.

CHAPTER 7

Emotional And Psychological Impact

Dealing With Emotions Before And After Surgery

Facing a hysterectomy, whether by medical necessity or personal choice, may elicit a broad range of emotions. It's acceptable to be nervous, worried, or relieved about the approaching treatment. Dealing with these emotions correctly may have a huge influence on your overall well-being and recovery.

Before surgery, it is critical to recognize and express your emotions. Tell your healthcare practitioner about any worries or anxieties you have. They may give useful information and assistance to ease your concerns. Additionally, speaking with others who have had a hysterectomy may provide insight and confidence.

During your recuperation, you may encounter an emotional rollercoaster. Allow yourself time to digest these emotions and be gentle with yourself. Allow yourself to relax and recover, both physically and emotionally. Taking part in things that offer you pleasure and relaxation will help you stay positive throughout this time.

Support Systems For Emotional Wellbeing

Having a solid support system may help you cope with the emotional problems of a hysterectomy. Surround yourself with friends, family, or support groups that can provide you encouragement, understanding, and practical help while you heal.

Communicate frankly with your loved ones about your emotions and wants. Please let them know how they can best help you at this time. Whether it's assisting with domestic tasks, giving transportation to medical visits, or just listening, having a trustworthy support network may help alleviate the emotional weight of surgery.

Addressing Issues With Body Image And Sexuality

A hysterectomy may cause changes in body image and sexuality that may need adjustment. It is normal to be self-conscious or uneasy about changes in your physical appearance or sexual function. However, you must understand that these modifications do not determine your value or femininity.

An open and honest conversation with your spouse about your worries and any changes you are feeling is essential. Together, you may find new methods to preserve closeness and deepen your relationship. If required, consulting with a healthcare physician or a sex therapist may assist in addressing particular sexual concerns after a hysterectomy.

Seeking Counseling Or Therapy As Needed

If you are having difficulty coping with the emotional repercussions of a hysterectomy, do not hesitate to seek expert assistance. Counseling or therapy may give you a safe and supportive setting in which to express your emotions, learn coping mechanisms, and gain perspective on your situation.

A skilled therapist can provide invaluable insight and support as you face the difficulties of surgery and recovery. Whether you're struggling with anxiety, sadness, or body image concerns, therapy may help you understand your feelings and discover healthy coping strategies.

Remember that asking for assistance when you need it is perfectly acceptable. Taking care of your mental well-being is equally as vital as looking after your physical health throughout the healing process.

CHAPTER 8

Fertility And Family Planning

Understanding The Fertility Implications Of Hysterectomy

When contemplating a hysterectomy, it is critical to understand the potential effect on fertility. A hysterectomy removes the uterus, but depending on the kind, it may also remove the cervix, fallopian tubes, and ovaries. This surgery presents a substantial obstacle to women who want to procreate in the future.

Pregnancy is impossible after a complete hysterectomy, which removes both the uterus and the cervix. This is because the uterus, which is where a fertilized egg implants and matures throughout pregnancy, no longer exists. However, if the ovaries continue to produce eggs, it may be feasible to conceive via alternate means such as surrogacy or gestational carriers.

Menopause is produced when the ovaries are removed (oophorectomy), which eliminates the potential for spontaneous pregnancy. Even if the ovaries are maintained, fertility decreases with age as ovarian function declines.

Exploring Alternative Options For Fertility Preservation

Women who want to keep their fertility but need a hysterectomy for medical reasons such as severe uterine fibroids or endometriosis have other choices to consider.

A myomectomy is a surgical treatment that removes fibroids while maintaining the uterus. This helps women to maintain their fertility while treating the underlying issue.

However, myomectomy may not be appropriate for all kinds of fibroids or in circumstances when the fibroids are very big or numerous.

Another alternative is uterine artery embolization (UAE), a minimally invasive technique that stops the blood flow to the fibroids, causing them to shrink. UAE maintains the uterus and may help relieve symptoms such as heavy menstrual flow and pelvic discomfort while not compromising fertility.

When conservative therapies are ineffective or impractical, fertility preservation procedures such as egg freezing or embryo cryopreservation may be used. These treatments include extracting and storing eggs or embryos for future use, enabling women to conceive following a hysterectomy using in vitro fertilization (IVF).

Discussing Family Planning Decisions With Your Partner And Healthcare Provider

Navigating the choice to have a hysterectomy and the consequences for family planning may be emotionally difficult. It is important to have open and honest conversations with your spouse and healthcare professional to explore your choices and make sound decisions.

Your healthcare professional may give essential information about the risks and advantages of hysterectomy, as well as other therapies and their effects on fertility. They can also advise you on fertility preservation procedures and send you to reproductive experts as required.

Involving your spouse in these talks is critical because they may give guidance and insight throughout the decision-making process. You may examine the benefits and drawbacks of each choice and decide which is best for your specific situation and family objectives.

Consider Adoption Or Other Family-Building Options

Following a hysterectomy, some women and couples may decide to parent via adoption or other family-building methods. Adoption allows you to give a caring home for a needy kid while also satisfying your ambition to be a parent.

There are many adoption options available, including domestic adoption, overseas adoption, and foster care adoption. Each option has unique criteria, protocols, and concerns, so it is important to do extensive study and obtain advice from adoption agencies or legal specialists.

Other possibilities for family formation, such as surrogacy and donor conception, may be viable alternatives to adoption.

Surrogacy is the employment of a gestational carrier to carry and deliver a child on behalf of the intended parents, while donor conception is the use of donated eggs, sperm, or embryos to become pregnant.

You may make educated choices about your fertility and family planning journey after a hysterectomy by evaluating all available options and discussing them honestly with your spouse and healthcare professional. Whether you want to seek pregnancy via alternative techniques or explore non-biological paths to motherhood, know that there are solutions available to help you achieve your goals of beginning or extending your family.

CHAPTER 9

Lifestyle Changes And Self-Care

Maintaining A Healthy Lifestyle Following A Hysterectomy

After having a hysterectomy, it is critical to emphasize your entire health and well-being. While the surgery tackles particular medical difficulties, keeping a healthy lifestyle thereafter may help you recover and improve your long-term health. Here's a thorough handbook that will help you navigate this path.

Regular Exercise Routine

Regular physical exercise is essential after a hysterectomy. However, it is critical to begin carefully and gradually increase the intensity and length of your exercises as your body recovers. Walking, swimming, and moderate yoga are all terrific options for beginners. These exercises boost circulation, build muscles, and enhance general health.

Balanced Diet

Nutrition is crucial to your rehabilitation. A balanced diet rich in fruits, vegetables, lean meats, and whole grains contains important elements for healing and general health. Adequate hydration is also important, so drink lots of water throughout the day.

Proper rest and recovery

Listen to your body and allow yourself plenty of time to rest and heal. Adequate sleep is required for healing, so aim for 7-9 hours of excellent sleep every night. Avoiding hard activities and taking time to rest will help your recuperation go more smoothly.

Regular medical check-ups

Schedule frequent follow-up consultations with your healthcare physician to track your progress and handle any issues or consequences that may emerge.

These meetings enable your doctor to check your recuperation and advise you on any lifestyle changes you should make after your hysterectomy.

Dietary Tips For Post-Hysterectomy Health

Maintaining a balanced diet is essential for your body's recovery and general well-being after a hysterectomy. Below are some dietary factors to bear in mind:

Adequate protein intake

Protein is required for tissue regeneration and muscular strength, making it particularly crucial during the recovery period. To promote healing and recuperation, include lean protein sources such as chicken, fish, tofu, beans, and lentils in your meals.

Fiber-rich foods

Constipation is a typical problem after a hysterectomy, so eating plenty of fiber-rich foods might help encourage regular bowel movements.

Include fruits, vegetables, whole grains, and legumes in your diet to guarantee appropriate fiber consumption.

Hydration

Proper hydration is vital for good health and healing. Aim to drink at least eight glasses of water every day, and restrict your consumption of caffeinated and alcoholic drinks, which may cause dehydration.

Balanced Nutrition

To improve your overall health and well-being, consume a balanced diet rich in nutrients. Include lots of fruits, vegetables, whole grains, lean meats, and healthy fats in your meals to ensure you're receiving the nutrients your body needs.

Pelvic Floor Exercise And Physical Therapy

Pelvic floor exercises and physical therapy may help women recover after hysterectomy by increasing pelvic floor strength, relieving discomfort, and promoting general pelvic health. Here's what you should know.

Importance of Pelvic Floor Health

The pelvic floor supports the pelvic organs and helps to maintain urine and bowel continence. Weakness or malfunction in the pelvic floor muscles may cause a variety of symptoms such as urine incontinence, pelvic organ prolapse, and discomfort.

Pelvic Floor Exercises

Pelvic floor exercises, often known as Kegel exercises, are used to contract and relax the pelvic floor muscles. These exercises serve to strengthen the pelvic floor muscles, increase pelvic organ support, and improve bladder and bowel control.

How To Perform Pelvic Floor Exercises

To conduct pelvic floor exercises, imagine yourself attempting to halt the flow of pee in the middle of the stream. Once you've discovered these muscles, contract them for 5-10 seconds before relaxing for the same time. Aim for 10-15 repetitions, many times each day.

Benefits of Physical Therapy

Physical therapy, in addition to pelvic floor exercises, may benefit women who have had a hysterectomy. A physical therapist may prescribe tailored exercises and procedures to treat particular pelvic floor disorders, increase mobility and flexibility, and relieve pain or discomfort.

Integrating Stress Management Techniques Into Everyday Life

Stress management is critical for general health and well-being, particularly after a major medical surgery such as a hysterectomy. Here are some useful ways to help you handle stress effectively:

Mindfulness & Meditation

Mindfulness and meditation may help relieve tension and promote relaxation. Take time each day to practice mindfulness exercises or guided meditation to help you relax and regain equilibrium.

Deep breathing exercises.

Deep breathing exercises may assist trigger the body's relaxation response, lowering tension and increasing sensations of peace. To assist relieve stress and tension, practice deep breathing exercises daily, with an emphasis on slow, deep breaths.

Regular exercise

Physical exercise is a great method to reduce stress and boost your mood. Regular exercise routines, such as walking, running, or yoga, may help relieve stress and increase overall health.

Healthy coping strategies

Find healthy methods to deal with stress, such as writing, spending time in nature, or participating in creative hobbies. Avoid employing unhealthy coping techniques, such as excessive alcohol intake or overeating, since they may be harmful to your health.

Seeking Support

If you are feeling overwhelmed, do not hesitate to seek help from friends, family, or a mental health professional. Talking to someone about your thoughts and experiences may give important support and perspective at difficult times.

CHAPTER 10

Moving Forward: Life After Hysterectomy

Reflecting On The Journey Of Hysterectomy

Reflecting on the hysterectomy process may be a very personal and emotional experience. For many people, having a hysterectomy is a major milestone in their life, accompanied by a variety of feelings such as relief, grief, and even dread. It's important to recognize and address these emotions as part of the healing process.

One component of contemplation is to evaluate why you decided to have a hysterectomy. Whether it was due to medical necessity, such as treating a chronic disease addressing reproductive health problems, or a personal choice for quality of life, understanding the motives may help people come to grips with their decision and go on with better clarity.

Furthermore, thinking about the physical and mental aspects of rehabilitation after a hysterectomy is critical. From the immediate recuperation phase after surgery to the gradual return to regular activities, each stage of the journey provides an opportunity for development and self-discovery. It is typical to have a variety of physical symptoms throughout recuperation, such as pain, exhaustion, and mood changes. Individuals may better navigate the rehabilitation process by admitting their experiences and seeking help when necessary.

Furthermore, focusing on the effects of hysterectomy on many parts of life, such as relationships, employment, and self-image, may be beneficial. While a hysterectomy may relieve symptoms and enhance the overall quality of life for many people, it can also create difficulties and changes. Individuals who recognize and confront these changes straight on might take proactive actions to adapt and prosper in their post-hysterectomy lives.

Setting Goals And Priorities For The Future

Setting future objectives and priorities is a crucial aspect of the post-hysterectomy recovery process. Whether it's resuming beloved hobbies, exploring new interests, or concentrating on personal development, having defined objectives may give direction and inspiration throughout the healing process.

One way to goal setting is to first determine the most significant aspects of one's life. This might encompass physical health, emotional well-being, relationships, job advancement, and personal growth. Individuals may direct their energy and attention toward activities and interests that are consistent with their beliefs and goals by prioritizing these areas.

It is also beneficial to establish both short-term and long-term objectives that are explicit, quantifiable, attainable, relevant, and time-bound. Short-term objectives might include progressively increasing physical activity levels, returning to employment or hobbies, or incorporating self-care activities like meditation or journaling. Long-term goals may include larger objectives such as enhancing general health and fitness, establishing rewarding relationships, or pursuing job improvements.

Additionally, goal-setting should be approached with flexibility and self-compassion. The healing process after a hysterectomy may be unpredictable, and patients may face setbacks or unforeseen problems along the road. Individuals who stay flexible and change their objectives as required may retain a feeling of progress and momentum in the face of adversity.

Embracing New Opportunities And Challenges

Embracing new chances and challenges is an important part of moving on after hysterectomy. While the choice to have surgery may have been motivated by particular health issues or situations, it also creates new opportunities and experiences.

One opportunity that exists with a hysterectomy is the possibility of increased health and well-being. For many people, a hysterectomy relieves severe symptoms like persistent pain, heavy bleeding, or pelvic discomfort, giving them a renewed feeling of vigor and independence. This enhanced physical resilience might provide possibilities to pursue hobbies and interests that were previously restricted by health issues.

Additionally, a hysterectomy might cause people to reconsider their objectives and ideals, resulting in personal development and self-discovery.

Whether it's reevaluating relationships, professional options, or lifestyle choices, the experience of having surgery and recovering may bring vital insights into what matters in life. Individuals who embrace these chances for self-reflection and development will come away with a stronger sense of clarity and purpose.

Of course, with fresh prospects come the usual difficulties and changes. Individuals may face a variety of emotional and practical challenges throughout recovery, including managing physical pain and exhaustion as well as negotiating changes in body image and sexuality. Individuals may create resilience and flexibility in the face of hardship by recognizing these problems and requesting assistance from healthcare experts, loved ones, and support groups.

Continue To Prioritize Self-Care And Overall Well-Being

Individuals recovering from a hysterectomy must maintain a focus on self-care and general well-being. While the recovery phase after surgery may need a focus on physical healing, committing to self-care is a lifelong path that covers all elements of health - physical, mental, and spiritual.

One part of self-care is to take care of one's physical health by regular exercise, a healthy diet, appropriate relaxation, and frequent medical checks. Gentle physical activity such as walking, swimming, or yoga may help the body repair and strengthen after a hysterectomy. Similarly, fueling the body with a well-balanced diet high in fruits, vegetables, whole grains, and lean meats will improve general health and vitality.

In addition to physical health, it is critical to emphasize emotional well-being via self-compassion, mindfulness, and stress reduction practices. Coping with the emotional consequences of a hysterectomy, including emotions of sadness, loss, or uncertainty, may need assistance from mental health specialists, support groups, or trusted loved ones. Individuals who acknowledge and handle these feelings healthily may create resilience and emotional well-being in the long run.

Furthermore, emphasizing spiritual well-being may provide people with a feeling of purpose, meaning, and connection in life. Nurturing the soul, whether via religious activities, meditation, nature walks, or artistic hobbies, may help you feel more fulfilled and satisfied overall. Individuals who include spiritual well-being activities in their every day lives may build a feeling of completeness and balance after a hysterectomy.

Conclusion

To summarize, knowing hysterectomy is critical for women contemplating this medical operation and those who assist them during the process. Throughout this thorough guide, we've covered all elements of hysterectomy, including its indications, types, risks, advantages, and alternatives.

First and foremost, it is critical to acknowledge that hysterectomy is a major medical procedure with consequences for physical, emotional, and psychological well-being. It is not a choice to be taken lightly, but rather after extensive consultation with healthcare specialists, evaluation of other therapies, and an understanding of personal circumstances and preferences.

For many women, a hysterectomy provides relief from painful gynecological disorders such as fibroids, endometriosis, persistent pelvic discomfort, and uterine prolapse. It may also be a life-saving surgery in the event of uterine malignancy or serious bleeding. However, it is critical to balance these advantages with the possible hazards and long-term repercussions, which include menopausal symptoms, sexual dysfunction, and psychological difficulties.

The kind of hysterectomy performed—total, subtotal, radical, or laparoscopic—is determined by many criteria, including the underlying ailment, the patient's health state, and the surgical aims. Each strategy has benefits and disadvantages, and the decision should be made individually based on thorough consideration and informed consent.

Alternative treatments for certain problems may also be offered, such as drugs, hormone therapy, less invasive surgeries, or careful waiting. These choices should be examined and discussed with healthcare practitioners to make an educated decision that is consistent with the patient's preferences and beliefs.

Communication and support are essential during the whole hysterectomy process. Patients should feel comfortable asking questions, expressing concerns, and seeking clarification regarding the treatment, recovery process, and possible results. Similarly, healthcare practitioners must give extensive preoperative counseling, perioperative treatment, and postoperative follow-up to improve patient outcomes and satisfaction.

Furthermore, emotional assistance from family, friends, support groups, or mental health experts may be beneficial in navigating the physical and emotional obstacles of hysterectomy. Open communication about worries, expectations, and coping methods may help people build resilience and adapt to life after a hysterectomy.

Finally, comprehending hysterectomy requires a comprehensive approach that considers medical, emotional, and social factors. Women may make educated choices regarding hysterectomy and face the path with confidence and resilience by educating themselves, receiving help from healthcare practitioners, and connecting with suitable support networks. Ultimately, the objective is to attain an enhanced quality of life and well-being, regardless of the route chosen for gynecological health and treatment.

THE END